Petals of Hope

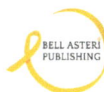

BELL ASTERI
PUBLISHING

Petals Of Hope

Brailynn Cumby

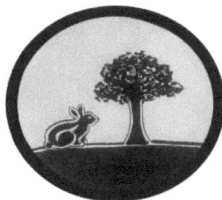

Published by Bell Asteri Publishing & Enterprises, LLC
209 West 2nd Street #177
Fort Worth TX 76102
www.bellasteri.com

Published in the United States of America

ISBN: 978-1-957604-86-2

table of Contents

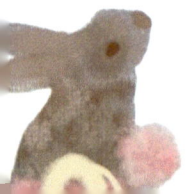

Dedication

To my family and my best friend Josie. You have been my solid rocks when I needed to express my feelings. Thank you for always supporting me, motivating me, and encouraging me to keep moving forward in the difficult times. You even laugh at my silly jokes and never find my ideas crazy. I love you.

To my Oncology Team, Fertility Specialists, Child Life Specialists, and Mrs. Allegra, thank you for your knowledge, patience, and encouragement when I was scared. I'm going to ring the bell!

This book is dedicated to all the families who have a child experiencing cancer. Together we share an adventure. You are never alone. We pray that every child is successful and that soon, no child will ever be diagnosed with cancer again.

"You are stronger than you think you are."
Fight on, Fighter – For King and Country.

It's been two weeks since I was diagnosed with cancer. I am so stuck on what I should do.

Should I laugh or should I cry?

Should I just do both?

Actually, right now I think I need to do both.

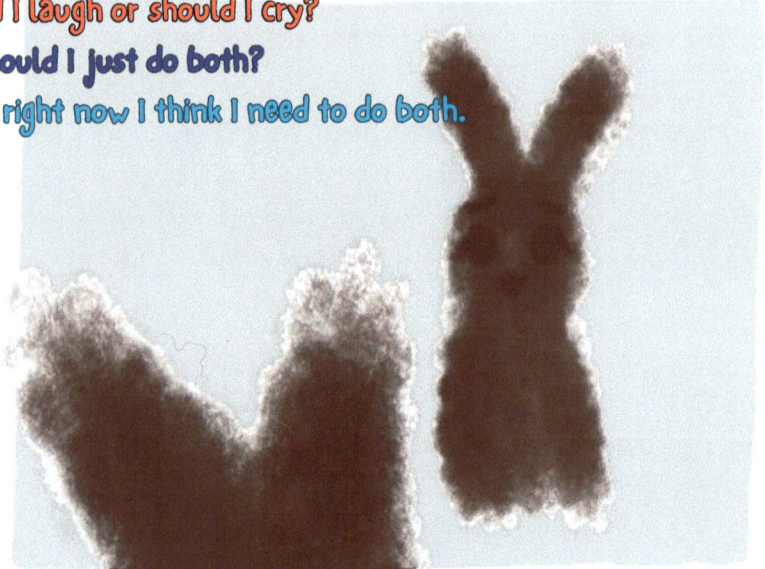

Who would've expected that the second I got home from school on a random Tuesday, I'd get told by my mother that I had cancer! What the heck is this? Really, right when my school life was going so well, too!

Are you seriously kidding me right now!

Well...at least it's not deadly. I think? It probably won't be. Yeah. I'm 100% sure that we caught it in time before it spread anywhere else.

My mother said that my first doctor's visit will be today. I'm a little nervous about what I'm going to have to do to get through this. I hope nothing is painful. I hate needles and surgeries so much.

The Enemy

the needle☹

My Reaction

?!!

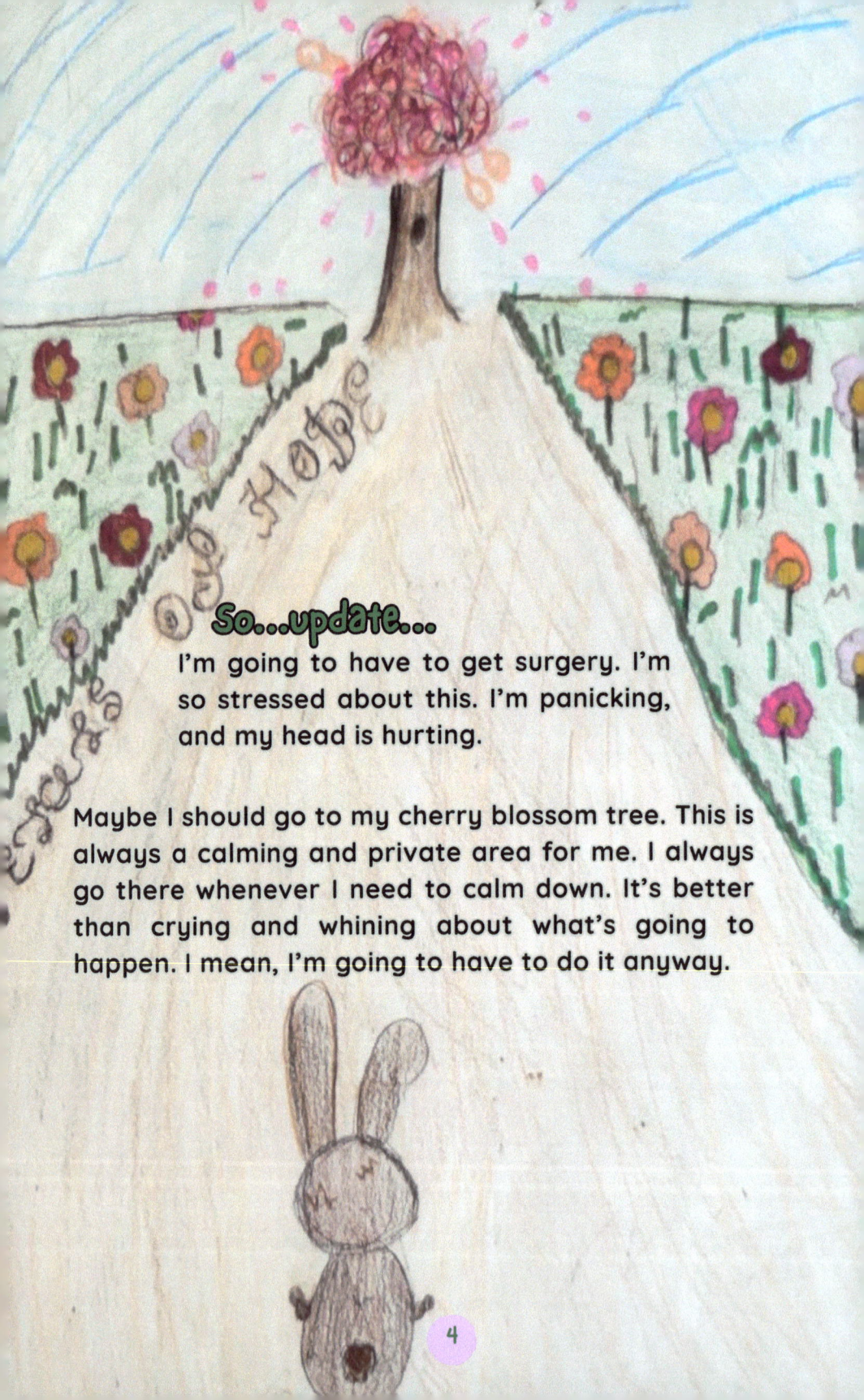

So...update...

I'm going to have to get surgery. I'm so stressed about this. I'm panicking, and my head is hurting.

Maybe I should go to my cherry blossom tree. This is always a calming and private area for me. I always go there whenever I need to calm down. It's better than crying and whining about what's going to happen. I mean, I'm going to have to do it anyway.

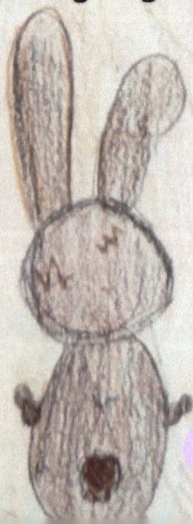

My mother bought me this tree back when I was around five or six. I have always loved cherry blossom trees, so she decided to buy me the seeds to plant it. I helped her plant it, and it took about five years for it to grow. Now I'm eleven, only eleven, going through this. I'm devastated but at the same time I know I'm strong.

For some reason that I cannot understand, no petals have ever fallen from this tree. I find it weird. All of the other trees around my tree lose their leaves and petals. Why not my cherry blossom tree? I'm not complaining because at least in the winter I get to look at a pretty bloomed tree. I just find it very strange. Hmmm... Mystery!

I sit back against my tree, get my notebook and pen, and start to write in it. I was gifted this notebook and so I'm going to use it to write about my journey through cancer. I can use my writings to help me get some of my emotions out that I can't really show at the hospital. If I get too emotional there, then I might mess up what the doctors are trying to do.

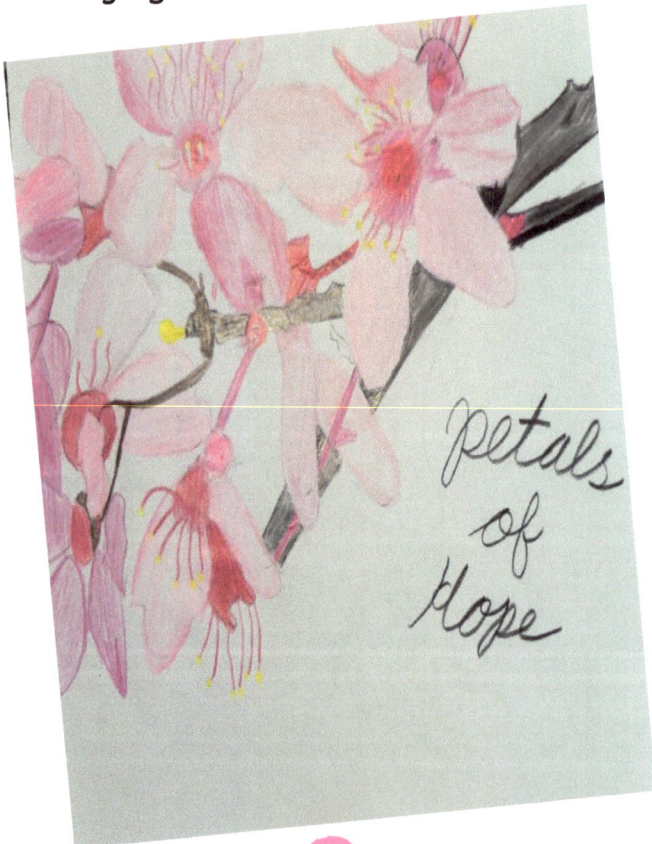

I write about how I'm scared for my surgery, how I'm sad about being diagnosed, how I'm feeling about my classmates, and how mad I am that it had to happen to me and no one else.

What did I do to get this? Am I going to survive?

The day of the surgery, my mother and I went to the hospital and had to go into the surgery waiting room. I'm terrified of what's going to happen.

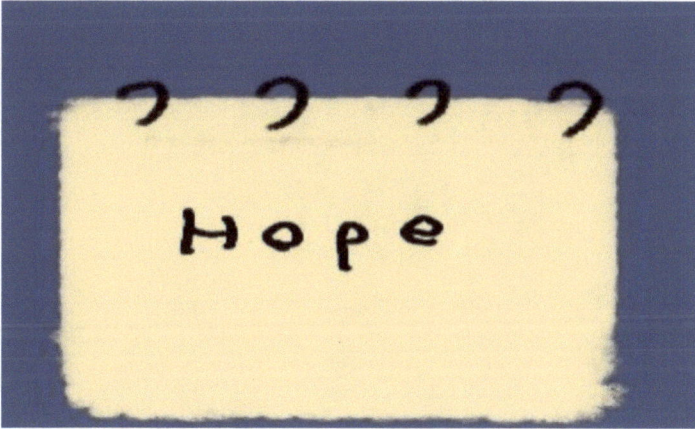

Once the nurse calls me back, they check my wristband and take my vitals.

I had to change into a hospital gown that I didn't like because the material is made like it's about to untie any second. Anyway, that's beside the point! Right?

So…after that, I had to go into a separate room, which is the "pre-operation room." Here we go!

My mom and I had to wait there for several minutes until the nurses came back with some supplies. I didn't pay attention to the supplies at first until I realized that the supplies were literally a needle and bandages. Yikes!

Just a warning from me to you kids: DO NOT do what I do on this next page because it is horrifically wrong....

ADVICE

DON'T DO WHAT I DID.

I started to PANIC and SCREAM!

Mind you, the nurses hadn't even got to me yet. The nurse said something like, "Hope, it's just an IV."

EXCUSE ME? Just an IV! Are you kidding me?

Have you seen the size of that needle? I stared at this nurse for so long that she eventually just grabbed my arm. I think you can guess what happened from there.

I screamed over and over again. It got even worse whenever she actually poked me. I sounded like a kid was getting absolutely tortured in that pre-operation room when it was just an IV!

The nurses had to hold me down. Yes. They had to call some other nurses who were specifically trained to help with kids. My own mother also had to help to hold me down. It was definitely not a pleasant experience.

SCORE

HOPE - 0

NEEDLE - 1

I JUST WANT A

PORT

So, after that wild incident, I just lay on the bed staring at the ceiling and waiting for them to give me my medicine to make me go to sleep. After I had calmed down, I kind of realized that I had embarrassed myself....and it wasn't so bad. It was actually really cringy! I bet you even cringed reading that, didn't you?

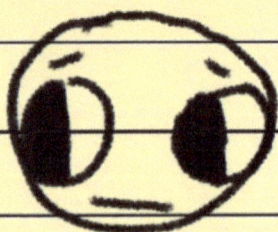

The surgery took a few hours, and I woke up in a different room. My back was in pain, and so was my neck. I remembered that they had removed my cancer and put a port in at the same time. Heads up! That was not a good idea to me at all. They would, of course, disagree.

Once I had fully awakened, my mom was sitting in a chair next to the bed. She told me, "You are so strong and beautiful, Hope. Don't you ever forget that." I kind of wondered why she suddenly said that. However, I was too out of it to even take in what she said before the nurse barges in and hits me with the news. She said, "You're going to have to stay the night."

"And you're enthusiastic about that? What?" I exclaimed. I must say that I was the most shocked I have been in the two weeks that I've been going through this.

My mother spoke up. She said, "Hope, it's only for one night. You get to go home in the morning. Calm down, baby."

That did give me some reassurance. However, I was still mad that they expected me to heal up, but then proceeded to put me on the most uncomfortable beds ever invented in the ENTIRE HISTORY OF HEALTHCARE! I mean, hey, at least it's not permanent.

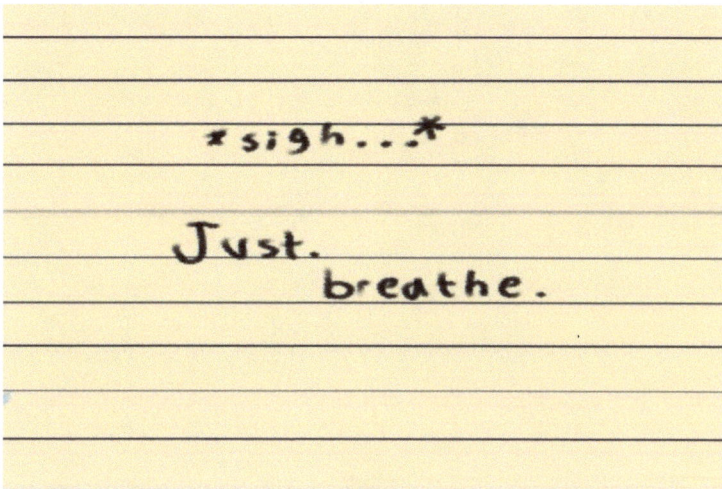

sigh...

Just.
        breathe.

We had to wait hours on top of hours for them to get me a room to stay in. And once they did, I'll tell you what, that room was so small the bed could barely even fit!

I was thinking to myself the entire time they tried to get me in, "There is absolutely no way they're putting me in this room out of all rooms. This is ridiculous."

They finally got me crammed into that room, but I was not happy with this. I was crying and complaining the entire night about wanting to go home. It didn't help that the nurses kept coming in and checking on me every single minute. Ugh! Just let me sleep in peace! Is that not what you want me to do?

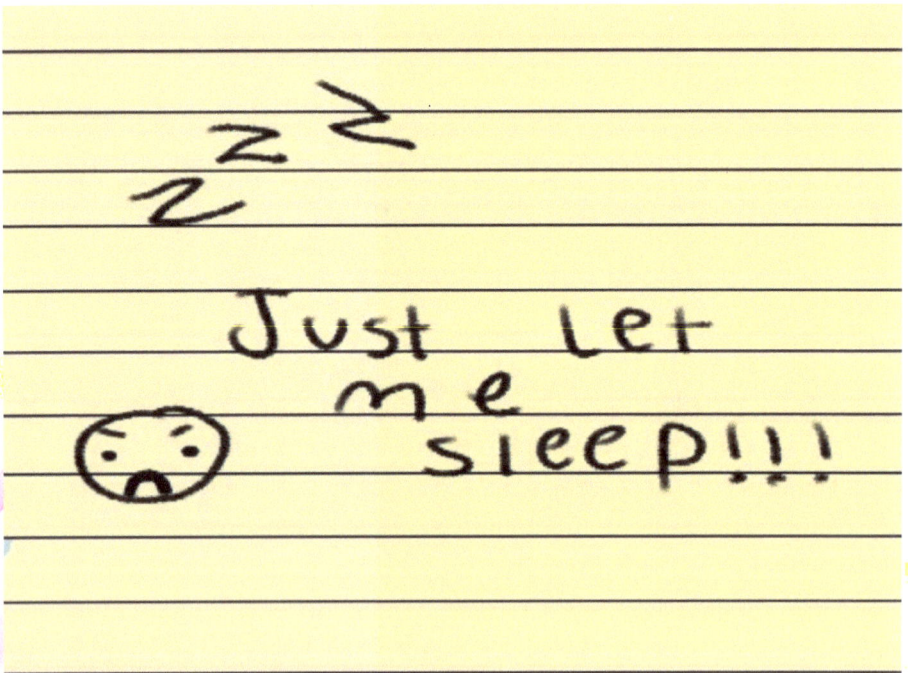

In the morning, I was finally able to go home. I was so happy that I could finally be able to sleep comfortably, in my own bed, without anyone or anything bothering me.

Quite honestly, the hospital stay wasn't so bad after all. It would've been better if I hadn't had any pain. However, as long as the cancer is gone now, then I think that I'm okay.

Score

Hospital - 0

Hope - 1

Made it through the nights! Gets easier EVERYTIME.

It took about a week for the surgery to heal up my incisions. I didn't go outside and write in my notebook during that time because I rested a lot in my bed. When I was feeling better, I went outside.

I walked down to my tree. I looked up at the tree and noticed that it was fully bloomed and had what I thought were all of its petals, as usual. I then looked at the ground and noticed that a single petal had actually fallen. I couldn't believe it. I immediately ran inside to get my basket.

Way back when the tree first bloomed, I bought this basket to collect the petals with, but as you know, the petals had never fallen! Seeing a petal fall from my special tree is so important to me. I ran back outside with my basket and picked up the petal right away.

I sat down with my basket, my pen, and my notebook. I began to write once again. This time, I wrote about how happy I was that a petal had fallen. I also wrote about how I'm one step closer to beating cancer. I got this. I know I'm strong.

I'm stronger than I think.

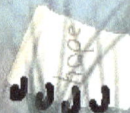

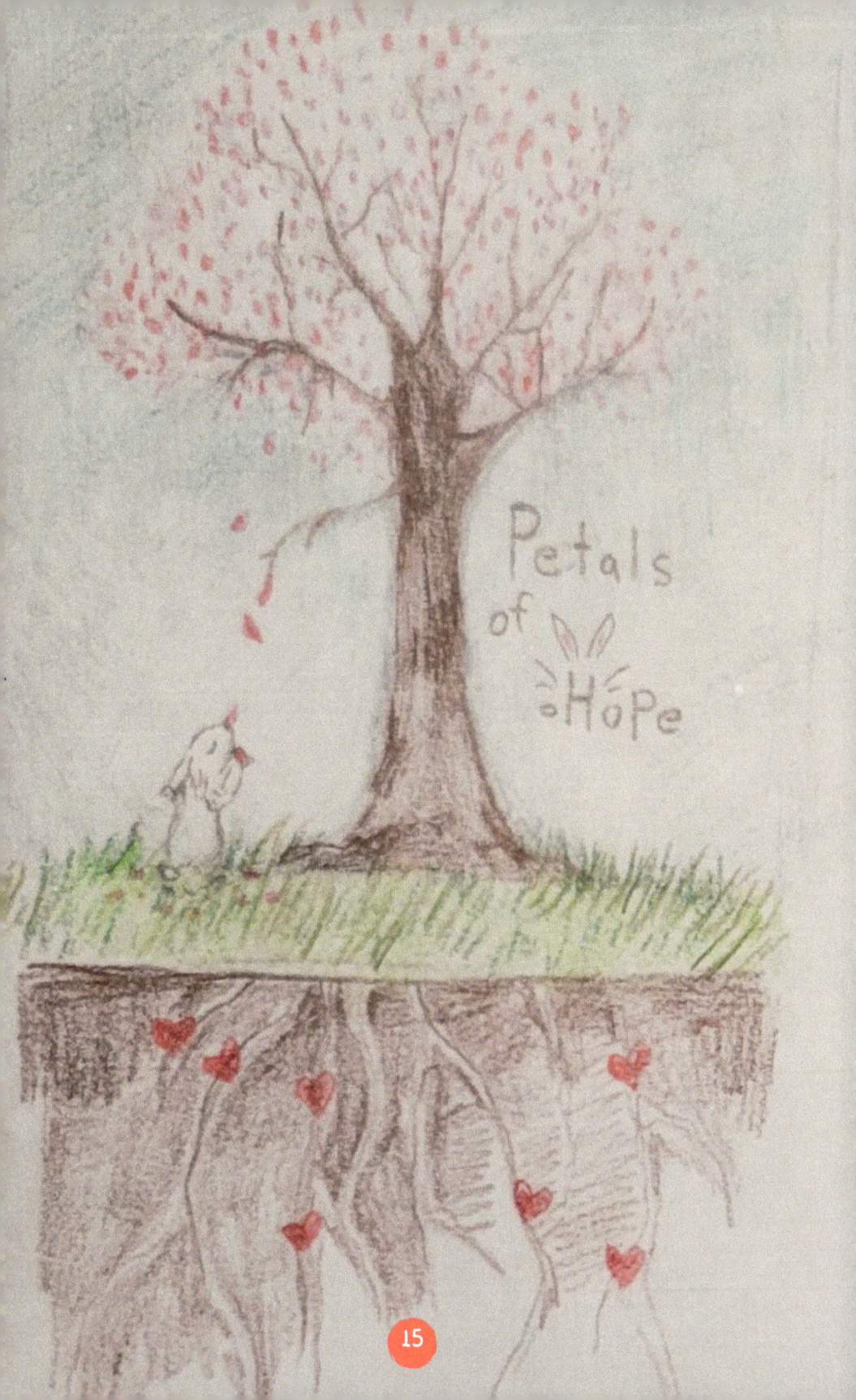

Petals
of
Hope

My mother told me that my first day of chemotherapy would be next week. I know that also means that it would be my first time accessing my port. I was downright terrified. Next week came around so fast. Faster than I had time to even prepare myself. I had some questions. How is this medication going to affect me?

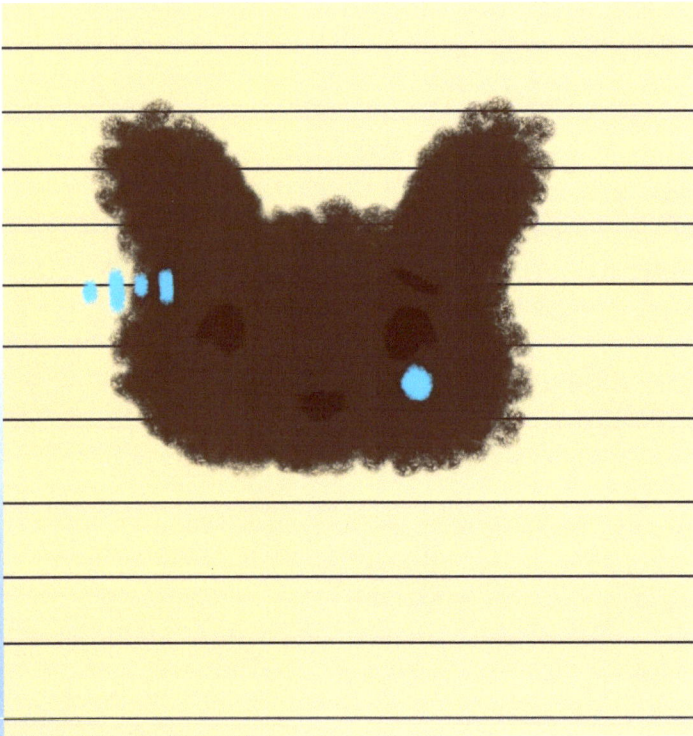

Am I going to lose all my fur?

What do I expect now?

I had to wake up very early in the morning just to get to the hospital on time, but it wasn't as early as I expected it to be. It was still pretty early, and I don't do early. Once we arrived, we started to walk to the waiting room to check in. When they called me back, the nurse told me I was getting a port access, and then she told me all of the steps required to do the port access. It sounded simple, really, a mask for germs, a lollipop swab to clean the skin, and a teenie tiny poke. Sure.

As before, that sure didn't go as planned. Again, I screamed and kicked. I'm pretty sure everyone in the hospital could hear me and the kid in the next room must have been traumatized. I apologize, but none of those things matter now.

ANXIETY

I'ts ok to ask questions.

PETALS OF HOPE

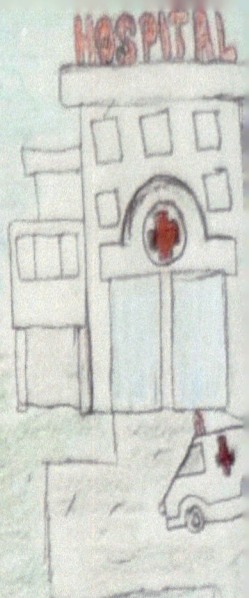

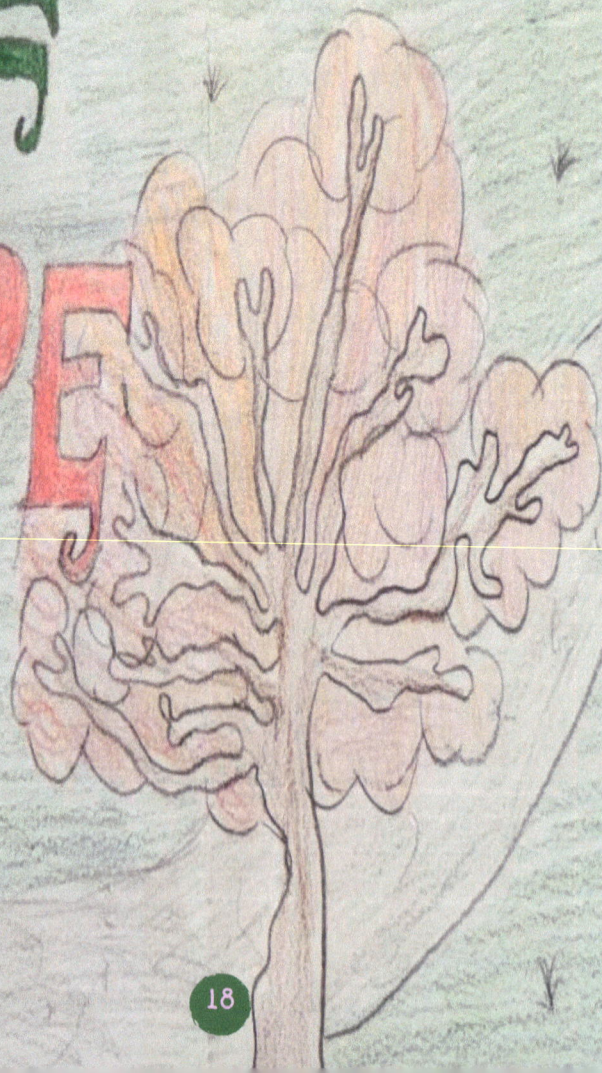

As long as I can get chemotherapy, I'm great. The nurses must deal with this a lot, as they were completely unbothered by my shenanigans.

I have to stay in the hospital for five days this time! Such a long time to be here, but I know what to expect this time. I won't be in pain this round as I have healed, so I expect that it should go better. At least I know that I'm not in here forever. I'll eventually get to go home. It will just take a few days.

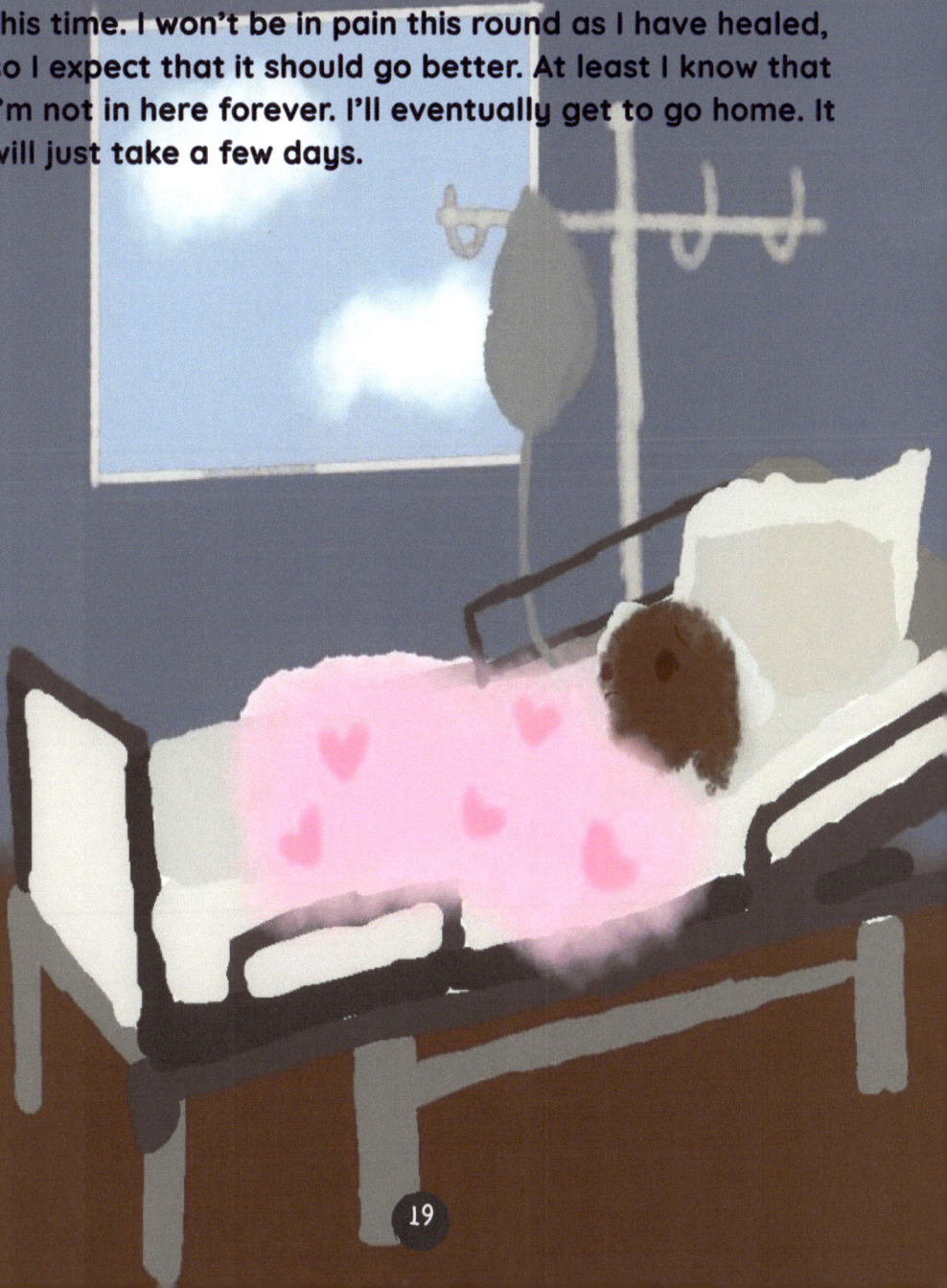

NOTE: I came up with a plan to overcome my port accesses

BE YOUR OWN ADVOCATE!

Told you it gets easier

didn't I?

As the five days went on, I would sleep a lot. Actually, I slept most of the time. When I was awake, I would draw, walk around the hospital, or play some games. It gets kind of repetitive, but it's really the only thing you can do whenever you're stuck in the hospital.

On the final night, I was so happy! I slept so much more easily. I got to go home as soon as the chemotherapy ended, and that was good because I didn't have to wait any longer.

The drive home took a while, but once I got back, I was finally able to rest. There's nothing like your own home and your own bed. In the morning, I grabbed my notebook and pen and went back to my tree.

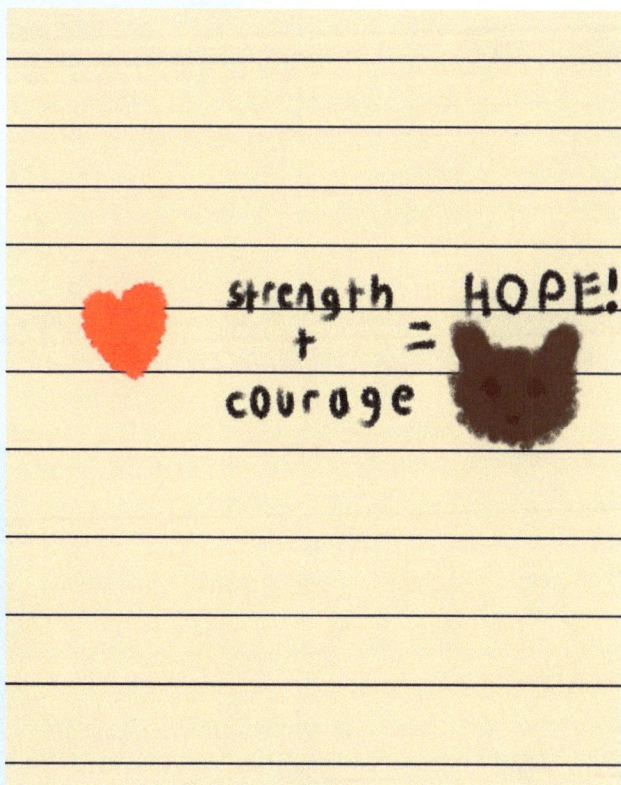

There are barely any more petals left on my tree. This makes me happy because my tree is finally going through changes. It's going to come back twice as beautiful. I just know it.

My notebook is very full now. It's full of my journey throughout this whole cancer thing. It expresses all of the feelings I've felt during this: happiness, sadness, and pain.

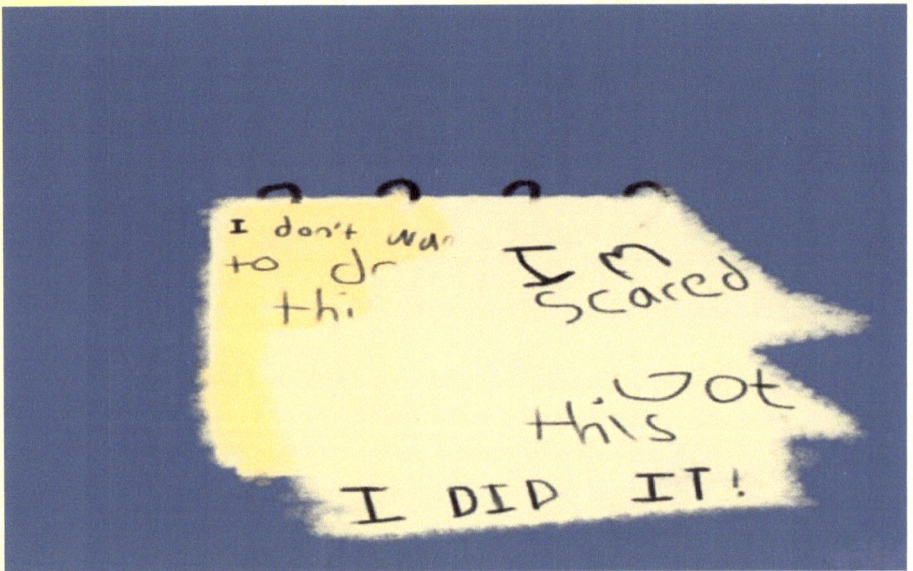

About two months later, I had to get some scans. These were special scans that look for signs of cancer throughout the body. They do these every several months, or so it seems. At the end of the day, my scan results came in. I am nervous and hopeful as to what they will say.

I beat cancer!!! Those special scans didn't see anything anywhere that looked as if it were cancer. Say it with me now:

"I BEAT CANCER!!!"

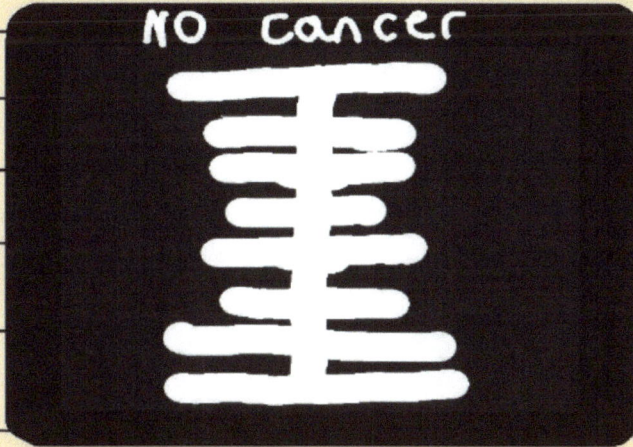

It was hard to believe that all of the fighting, all of the medicine, and all of the new adventures that I've never been through before helped to fight the cancer away. It seemed like such a hard journey in the beginning, but now I feel like I can see the end, and I'm going to be alright.

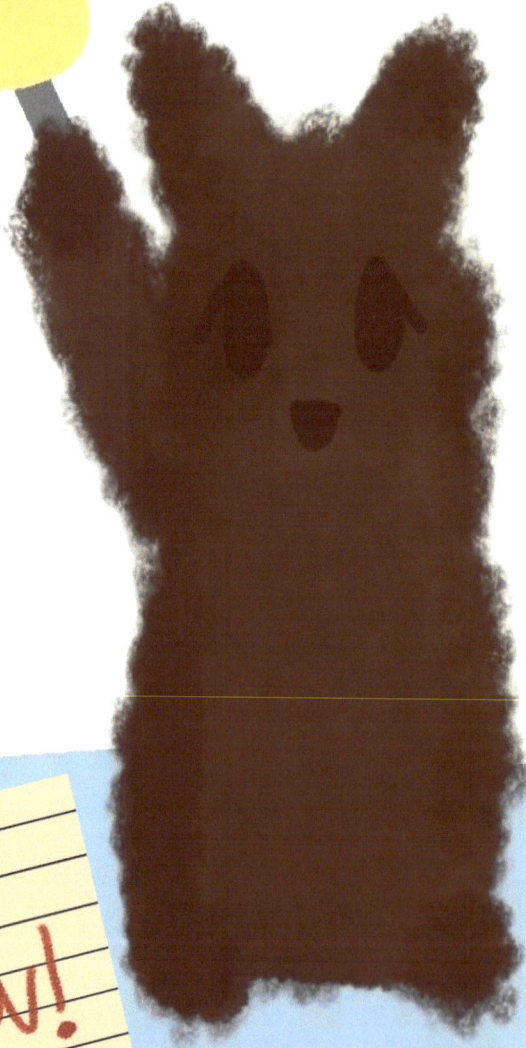

The drive home felt bright. There were no worries, no fears, and no sadness anymore. My illness is gone. I'm finally healed. I know that I will have more rounds of chemotherapy to finish the schedule. I will also have scheduled scans for a really long time, but it will all be worth it.

Once we got home, I couldn't wait to write in my notebook. As I went outside to sit under my tree, I noticed that all of the petals were gone. My tree has no more petals left. Why? Hmmm...mystery.

I realized something in that moment. The tree is just like me. My tree has no more leaves, and my body has no more cancer or fur now. The medicines caused my fur to fall out. Guess what? I'm still the same person now, just like my tree is the same tree. It will take a while for my body to bounce back from the medicine, and it will take a while for my tree to grow back its petals. I just KNOW that we will both come back twice as beautiful as we were before. There's beauty in changes.

We are stronger than we know.

Honorable Mentions

Some of the artwork in this book was provided by participating students at Flat Rock Middle School in North Carolina. This art project was done in collaboration with two teachers, Mr. Lee (Art) and Mr. Byrd (Social Studies). Students whose artwork was featured in the story and one logo that will be used for inspiration on a future clothing project were provided with a monetary prize and a special day in class for their donations and cooperation. I want to say a big thank you to the participants. I truly felt so much love and support from everyone involved. I hope my readers will enjoy the art pieces as much as I have.

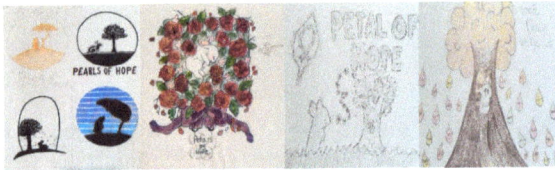

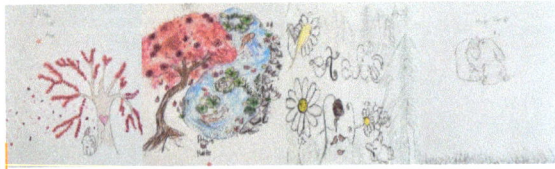

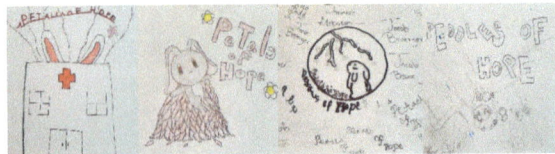

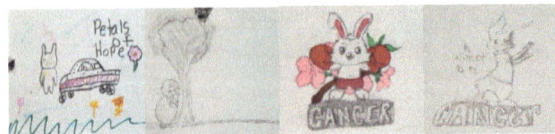

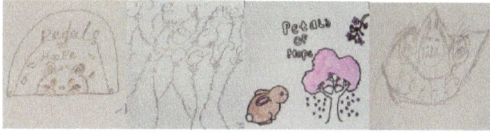
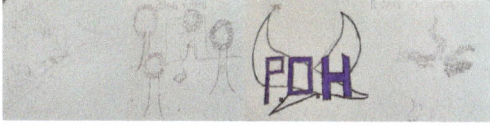
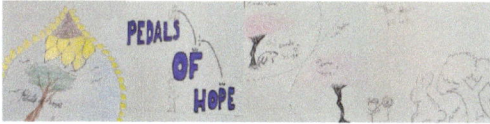
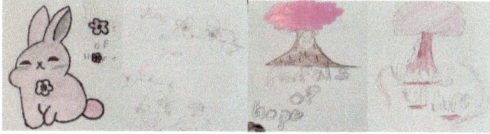
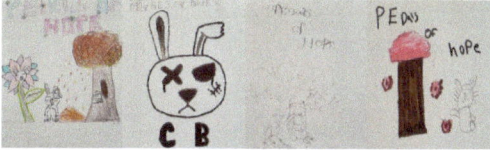
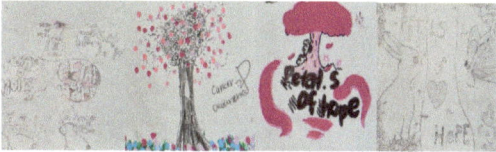
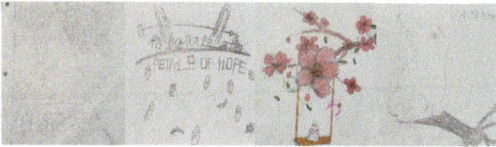
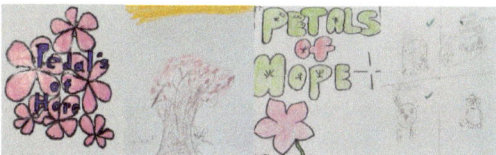

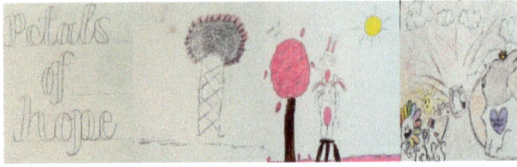
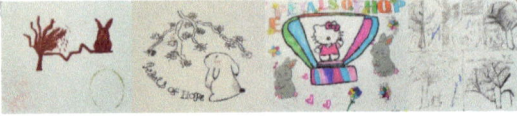
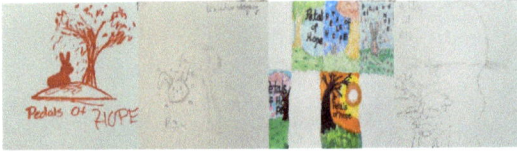
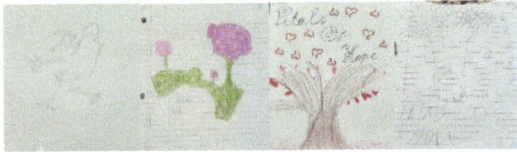
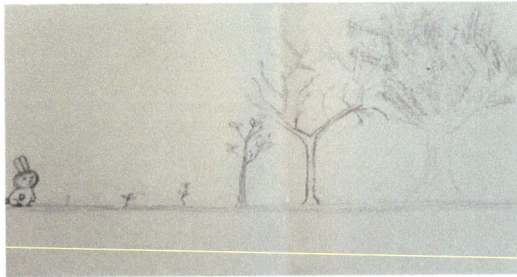

About the Author

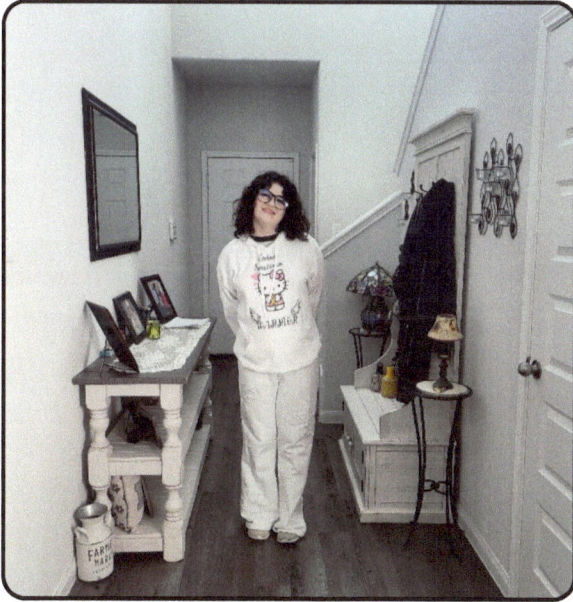

Brailynn Cumby was born on March 28th, 2013, in Springfield, Missouri. She lived in Missouri until 2023, when she moved to Conroe, Texas. She is currently a 7th grader.

Brailynn was always an active child, and she exhibited creativity from an early age. She was always doing cosplays and drawing. Along with her artistic creativity, she loved sewing, acting, music, dance, and anything "Hello Kitty."

She was diagnosed with a benign cyst in May 2024. However, the cyst was removed and biopsied in September 2024 after it had grown rapidly in size. The results showed that Brailynn had a type of cancer called Ewing's Sarcoma. PET scans and CT/MRIs confirmed that cancer was present. The cancer was localized in the soft tissue of her back, but she needed a second surgery to achieve negative margins.

Brailynn then underwent fertility treatments to preserve her eggs for the future before beginning the standard treatment of VDC/IE chemotherapy. In March 2025, Brailynn's PET/CT/MRI scans showed no evidence of disease, followed by maintenance chemotherapy. In September 2025, Brailynn rang the bell proclaming she was cancer-free at the **Fight like a Kid** event at KMS Speedway and Texas Children's Hospital.

During her chemotherapy, Brailynn desired to help other kids by sharing her experience. She began writing in a journal about her feelings, and eventually this led to her writing this book for kids. It was originally published in Spring 2025 and then republished in early 2026 as a second edition.

She often complained that the hospital gowns were uncomfortable and the chemotherapy shirts on the market failed to have a pocket to hold her phone and earbuds while she was getting her treatments. She also didn't like that the shirts kept falling into the sterile field while trying to access her chemo port. This led her to design her own chemotherapy shirt that addressed the issues. She recently had a prototype made. Brailynn has already gotten her first customer, and she will expand her business into an online store. She is in the process of creating her brand.

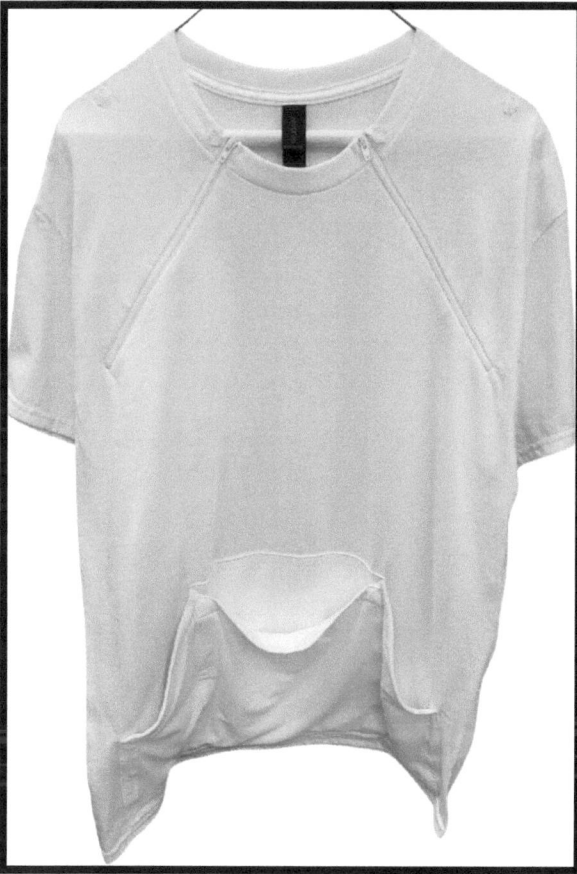

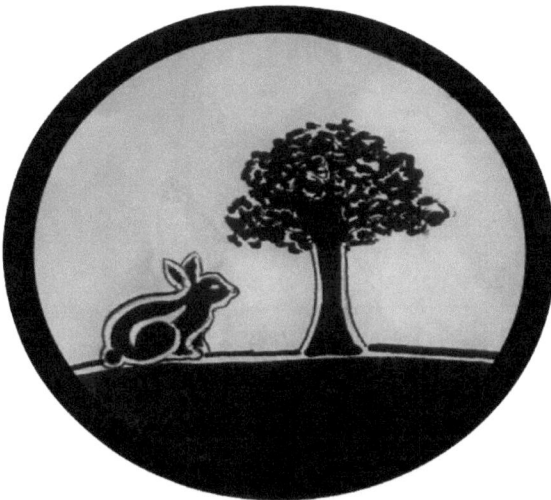

Petals Of Hope

www.ingramcontent.com/pod-product-compliance
Lightning Source LLC
Chambersburg PA
CBHW041303290326
41931CB00032B/34